How-to Guide: Viagra

Pills for Men – Acting Fast, Get and Stay Hard, Long Lasting Erection, Guaranteed Mind-blowing Climax

Dr. Ida Lacy

DISCLAIMER

For your specific needs, it is imperative that you speak with your doctor. Before beginning any new fitness program, you should seek the advice and knowledge of your own physician. This book is not meant to take the place of the cost-effective medical advice from a qualified physician.

Table of Content

Chapter One

Cialis

Overview

Sildenafil citrate, known by its popular brand name Viagra, has played a transformative role in the field of male sexual health by revolutionizing the treatment of erectile dysfunction. However, its impact extends far beyond its ability to facilitate erections. This remarkable pharmaceutical agent has shown remarkable effectiveness in managing various cardiovascular conditions, such as pulmonary arterial hypertension. It is worth mentioning that Revatio, another name for the same active ingredient, Sildenafil citrate, has also been widely used in medical practice. The versatility of this medication has had a profound positive impact on the quality of life and overall satisfaction of countless individuals all over the globe.

Initially conceived as a groundbreaking medical breakthrough targeting the pressing concern of hypertension, Viagra has undergone a remarkable metamorphosis, solidifying its standing as a universally recognized and predominantly employed remedy for the pervasive problem of male impotence. Since its inception, Viagra has amassed an impressive repertoire of achievements in enhancing the overall contentment and gratification derived from male sexual encounters.

The effectiveness and duration of Viagra can vary based on various factors. While it usually takes around thirty minutes for the effects to become noticeable, this timeframe can be influenced by multiple variables. These include your diet, overall health, concurrent usage of other medications, pre-existing health conditions, and various other factors. It is important to consider these elements as they can impact both the onset of Viagra's effects in your body and how long it remains effective.

How Viagra Works

Erectile dysfunction, also referred to as impotence, is a medical condition that interferes with an individual's ability to achieve or maintain an erection that is considered satisfactory for sexual activities. This problem arises from a breakdown in the complex communication system between the brain and the nervous system, which ultimately leads to insufficient blood flow to the specialized chambers within the penis called the corpus cavernosa. These chambers, consisting of sponge-like tissue, play a crucial role in the process of becoming engorged with blood and facilitating an erection. Consequently, when the nerves fail to transmit the appropriate signals, it disrupts this vital mechanism and presents obstacles in attaining a firm and long-lasting erection.

When an individual takes an oral tablet of Viagra, it usually takes between thirty to sixty minutes for the medication to start working and achieve the desired therapeutic effects. This timeframe allows the drug to be absorbed by the body and begin interacting with the necessary biological processes that improve blood flow. It is important to note that the exact time for Viagra to take effect may vary slightly among individuals due to factors like metabolism and overall health. However, once Viagra starts working, it creates optimal conditions for a more satisfying sexual experience by enhancing blood circulation specifically in the penis. Viagra is designed to treat erectile dysfunction by significantly improving blood flow to the penis. Its mechanism involves relaxing the walls of blood vessels, which in turn promotes a smoother blood flow to the parts of the penis responsible for achieving an erection. By enhancing blood flow, Viagra helps individuals achieve and maintain a firm erection.

In order for Viagra to effectively bring about the desired results, it is crucial to comprehend that it does not initiate an erection by itself. The presence of sexual stimulation is imperative for Viagra to induce the intended effects. Nonetheless, it has been noted that individuals who are in a state of relaxation and tranquility may potentially experience the effects of Viagra at an earlier stage.

The main objective of Viagra is to help individuals who struggle with erectile dysfunction by improving their ability to achieve and maintain erections. Its aim is to boost sexual performance and stamina for those who experience this issue. However, if you do not experience erectile dysfunction, there are other treatment choices available that may better cater to your individual needs and preferences.

The duration of Viagra's effects usually ranges from two to three hours before diminishing, but this timeframe can be influenced by various factors such as dosage, metabolism, and environmental factors. There are instances where the effects of Viagra can last up to five hours or more. Individuals with erectile dysfunction may need to wait approximately one hour before experiencing the desired effects of Viagra, and it is recommended to take the medication at least four hours before engaging in sexual activities.

The frequency of experiencing erections while taking Viagra can vary among individuals due to differences in their body's metabolic processes, leading to some people encountering this particular side effect more frequently than others.

While Viagra may not be effective in sustaining an erection post-ejaculation, it does allow individuals to prolong their sexual encounters for as long as the medication is effective. It is important to keep in mind that there may be a required waiting period between achieving orgasm and being able to achieve another erection.

In spite of the multitude of advantages offered by Viagra,

there are certain concerns that it
does not adequately tackle.

✓ Premature ejaculation,
which is a common problem
of achieving orgasm too
quickly, can present a
significant challenge for
individuals. To effectively
address this issue, it is
recommended to explore
different strategies or seek
out specific treatments
designed to address
premature ejaculation.

✓ In addition to the points
mentioned above, there is
another issue that Viagra
cannot fully address, which

11

is the sensation of tiredness that arises during sexual activity. Nevertheless, there are alternative tactics that can be employed to overcome this concern. One effective method is to concentrate on enhancing your overall stamina and endurance levels. This can be accomplished through various means, such as engaging in regular physical activity and maintaining a healthy lifestyle. Additionally, incorporating caffeine into your daily regimen can offer an additional surge of energy.

By implementing these actions, individuals have the potential to alleviate feelings of fatigue and enhance their overall sexual encounter.

✓ If you are facing a decrease in sexual desire or a low libido, depending only on Viagra might not be the most effective solution. It is strongly recommended to explore lifestyle modifications or contemplate therapy to tackle the underlying causes of this decline in your sexual drive. By embracing a holistic approach and addressing the fundamental issues, you have the opportunity to revive and enhance your sexual desire in a more enduring and gratifying manner.

The duration for which Viagra remains in the body tends to vary from individual to individual, typically ranging from two to three hours. Nevertheless, in certain instances, it might persist for as long as five to six hours, contingent upon the speed at which an individual's metabolism operates. Moreover, the length of time Viagra stays in the body is influenced by the dosage taken. To illustrate, a smaller dose of 25mg generally dissipates more rapidly, whereas a higher dose of 100mg may require a significantly longer period to be entirely eliminated from the system.

If you discover that Viagra is not working as quickly as you had hoped, it may be beneficial to engage in activities such as self-stimulation or intimate play to enhance arousal. However, it is crucial to bear in mind that if these methods fail to produce the desired outcome within thirty minutes, it is vital not to exceed the recommended daily dosage provided by your healthcare professional. Taking an excessive amount of Viagra can result in a condition called priapism, which involves a long-lasting and painful erection lasting for more than four hours. This can be detrimental to the health of the penis since the blood trapped in the organ lacks oxygen and may cause tissue damage.

In the event that this particular scenario arises, it is of utmost importance and highly recommended that you expeditiously and resolutely pursue urgent medical assistance without any hesitation or procrastination. It is absolutely essential to prioritize and safeguard your general health and welfare by taking prompt measures and reaching out to proficient healthcare practitioners. By doing so, you will guarantee receiving the essential medical attention needed for your recuperation, thereby avoiding any avoidable delays.

Chapter Two

Viagra Usage

The dosage of Viagra that is recommended varies based on the specific condition it is being used to treat, whether it is erectile dysfunction or pulmonary arterial hypertension.

Viagra, a well-known medication, is widely used by men facing the frustrating issue of erectile dysfunction as a reliable pharmaceutical solution. It can be easily obtained in the market in the form of distinctive blue tablets that bear a resemblance to diamonds. These tablets are carefully manufactured to cater to a range of strengths, ranging from 25mg to 100mg, enabling men to find the exact dosage that suits their specific needs and helps them overcome the challenges they face in attaining and sustaining an erection. It is crucial to emphasize the utmost importance of strictly adhering to the recommended dosage guidelines, which state that only one pill should be consumed within a 24-hour period. By diligently following this guidance, users can ensure that they optimize the effectiveness of Viagra and attain the desired outcomes in their sexual encounters. To further enhance the medication's potency, it is advisable to consume the pill approximately 30 minutes to an hour prior to engaging in any sexual activity. This allows ample time for the medication to take effect and significantly enhance the overall sexual experience.

Revatio, which is also known as Viagra, is a medication that comes in the shape of circular tablets with a smooth outer layer. This drug is primarily prescribed to individuals who suffer from pulmonary arterial hypertension, a medical condition that affects the blood vessels in the lungs. To effectively control and treat this condition, healthcare providers usually recommend patients to take a 20mg tablet of Revatio three times a day. It is crucial for patients to adhere to this dosage regimen consistently and punctually in order to achieve the best possible results.

If you ever believe that you have ingested too much Viagra, it is vital that you take immediate action by reaching out to a healthcare professional or contacting the Poison Control Center nearest to you. Exceeding the prescribed amount of this medication can have serious consequences and should not be taken lightly. Therefore, it is imperative that you seek urgent medical help if you have any suspicion or sign of an overdose.

There are a variety of signs and symptoms that may suggest someone is experiencing an overdose, with a wide range of potential indicators that could be present.

- ✓ Vomiting
- ✓ Diarrhea
- ✓ Blindness
- ✓ Blurred or distorted vision
- ✓ Damage to the optic nerve, called optic neuropathy
- ✓ Prolonged and painful erection

- ✓ Swelling of the optic nerve, called papilledema
- ✓ Rapid heartbeat, called tachycardia
- ✓ The breakdown of muscle tissue is called rhabdomyolysis.

Although not common, death is also a possible result.

Having a discussion with your healthcare provider before deciding to use Viagra or any other medication for erectile dysfunction is extremely important. This step should not be taken lightly or disregarded in any way. Seeking professional medical advice is crucial in order to be well-informed and make the best choices for your health and overall well-being. Your doctor possesses the necessary expertise and knowledge to thoroughly assess your individual circumstances, taking into account various factors such as your overall health, existing medical conditions, and potential interactions with other medications you may be taking. They can provide personalized advice and recommendations tailored specifically to your needs, helping you navigate the potential benefits and risks associated with the use of Viagra or similar medications. It is essential to remember that your healthcare provider's guidance and expertise are invaluable when it comes to decisions that could impact your sexual health and overall quality of life. Do not hesitate to schedule a consultation to address any concerns or questions you may have regarding this topic.

There are specific medications, like nitroglycerin and other nitrates, that have been developed to effectively address heart conditions. These medications have shown to offer significant advantages for individuals dealing with cardiac problems. Nevertheless, it is crucial to acknowledge that combining these medications with Viagra, a well-known drug employed to treat erectile dysfunction, can potentially result in hazardous outcomes. One of the risks associated with this combination is a significant decrease in blood pressure, a consequence that should not be taken lightly or disregarded.

Chapter Three

Factors Affecting Viagra

There are many factors that can potentially affect how effective and long-lasting the effects of Viagra are, and these factors may vary depending on the unique circumstances of each person.

Diet

Consuming a large or fatty meal prior to using Viagra can hinder the body's ability to process the medication and may hinder achieving an erection. On the other hand, this can also extend the duration of the medication's effectiveness as it is metabolized with the meal. Conversely, taking

Viagra without eating can result in faster onset of its effects.

Alcohol

The male reproductive organ's blood flow is negatively affected by the consumption of alcohol, which results in difficulties in achieving and maintaining an erection. It is important to note that consuming excessive amounts of alcohol alongside Viagra greatly increases the risk of experiencing harmful side effects, surpassing the recommended maximum intake of two units. These side effects can further impede an individual's ability to achieve a satisfactory erection.

Age

As individuals age, it is common for their metabolism to gradually decline. This phenomenon is particularly evident among males aged 65 and older, who may undergo a slightly prolonged period of decreased metabolic rate.

Dosage

The duration of Viagra's presence in your system is determined by the amount you consume. Generally, opting for a higher dosage will prolong its benefits and yield superior outcomes. Nonetheless, it is essential to consult with your healthcare provider to determine the appropriate dosage for your specific requirements, as consuming excessive amounts may not be safe or recommended.

Medications

To ensure that there are no complications or interactions between clarithromycin (Biaxin), erythromycin (Ery-Tab), ciprofloxacin (Cipro), and Viagra, it is strongly advised to consult your primary care doctor. Seeking guidance from a healthcare professional will help you prioritize your well-being and make informed choices about your medication schedule.

Psychological State

Anxiety, nervousness, stress, or depression can have a substantial impact on how your body reacts to sexual stimulation, which could potentially diminish the duration or efficacy of Viagra.

Health

There are several pre-existing medical conditions that can affect how long and how well Viagra works. People with conditions like diabetes, multiple sclerosis (MS), or atherosclerosis (a condition where fatty deposits build up in blood vessels) may experience less effectiveness from Viagra, causing the effects to last for a shorter time. Additionally, specific liver or kidney conditions may cause Viagra to stay in the body for longer periods as the body needs more time to process and eliminate the medication.

Chapter Four

Is Viagra Safe?

In most cases, when used appropriately, Viagra is generally considered to be safe for consumption. Nevertheless, it is crucial to recognize that the utilization of this medication can lead to various negative consequences. It is imperative to understand and acknowledge the potential hazards that may arise from taking Viagra.

The results of the clinical trial have provided valuable insights into the numerous adverse reactions frequently experienced by individuals taking Viagra. These findings highlight the potential risks associated with this medication, as a range of side effects have been consistently observed. Although not an exhaustive compilation, some of the commonly documented negative effects include.

- ✓ Visual impairments encompass a variety of conditions that affect an individual's capacity to see or comprehend visual information.
- ✓ Digestive problems, including indigestion, which entails difficulties in

breaking down and digesting food, may occur.

✓ Nasal congestion, also referred to as a congested or obstructed nose, is a condition that arises when the nasal passages become swollen or inflamed.

✓ Photophobia is a condition that is characterized by a heightened sensitivity to light.

✓ Headaches

Besides the things we already talked about, there are some other things that might happen to a person. These things are called side effects and they can make a person feel different or not as good as usual.

- ✓ Sudden loss of hearing.
- ✓ Ventricular arrhythmia, a medical condition, is identified by irregular heartbeats that arise from the lower chambers of the heart.
- ✓ A heart attack, also known as a myocardial infarction.
- ✓ Increased pressure inside the eye, known as intraocular pressure, can result in various eye-related issues.
- ✓ Priapism is a rare condition characterized by a long-

lasting and painful erection. This medical issue is caused by blood getting trapped in the penis, leading to discomfort. While priapism is not common, individuals experiencing it may feel scared and disturbed.

In exceedingly rare instances, a small cluster of individuals who have consumed Viagra have reported encountering an unusual visual phenomenon known as Cyanopsia, wherein they perceive their surroundings with a subtle blue hue. It is imperative to emphasize that this occurrence is highly uncommon and does not impact the majority of users. It is also crucial to underscore that in highly exceptional scenarios, the utilization of Viagra has been associated with a potential risk of developing a condition referred to as nonarteritic anterior ischemic optic neuropathy, which results in harm to the optic nerve. However, it is essential to highlight that the probability of experiencing these adverse effects is extremely minimal, and the overwhelming majority of individuals who employ Viagra do not encounter any complications with their eyesight.

Viagra has the potential to cause a rare occurrence where individuals may experience sudden vision loss due to its ability to restrict blood flow to the optic nerve. However, it is important to note that this harmful effect is not commonly seen and primarily affects those who already have medical conditions such as diabetes, high cholesterol, pre-existing eye disorders, heart problems, or high blood pressure.

It is crucial for individuals with HIV who are taking protease inhibitors to speak with their doctor before using Viagra. This is important because protease inhibitors can increase the risk of negative side effects from Viagra and make them more severe. Therefore, it is recommended that individuals in this group limit their Viagra intake to no more than 25mg within a 48-hour period. Seeking advice from a healthcare provider is essential to ensure the safe and appropriate use of Viagra for those managing HIV and protease inhibitor treatment. This precaution is necessary because protease inhibitors can heighten the likelihood of experiencing adverse effects and worsen their intensity. Therefore, it is advised for individuals in this specific category to restrict their use of Viagra to 25mg over a 48-hour period. By adhering to this guidance and consulting their doctor, individuals can ensure responsible use of Viagra while effectively managing their HIV and protease inhibitor treatment.

In addition to the points mentioned above, it is extremely important for individuals who have been prescribed alpha-blockers to exercise great caution and vigilance when it comes to the timing of their Viagra consumption. The timing of these medications must be carefully controlled and coordinated, ensuring a significant time gap of at least four hours before or after taking alpha-blockers. This precautionary measure is absolutely essential in order to minimize the risks associated with a significant drop in blood pressure, which could potentially lead to severe and harmful health complications. Therefore, it becomes crucial to prioritize and give the utmost attention to the precise coordination and arrangement of these medications when using them together.

Chapter Five

Those to Avoid Viagra

Viagra is a medication intended specifically for men who are 18 years of age or older. It is important to understand that this medication may not be safe or appropriate for everyone. It is crucial for women and individuals under the age of 18 to use caution and avoid using this medication.

People who have had an allergic reaction to Viagra or any other medication are advised to avoid using it. This includes individuals who have previously had negative reactions to the drug and should be careful when contemplating its future use. It is crucial for this group to understand the potential dangers linked to taking Viagra and to seek guidance from a healthcare professional before starting any new medication routine. By taking proactive steps to steer clear of possible allergic reactions, they can effectively prevent severe health issues and safeguard their overall health and welfare.

- ✓ Individuals who are experiencing liver and heart problems.
- ✓ People who have recently had a stroke or heart attack.

- ✓ Individuals afflicted with kidney disease.
- ✓ There are numerous individuals who experience rare genetic eye disorders or have inherited conditions leading to retinal degeneration.
- ✓ Individuals experiencing low blood pressure are also known as having hypotension.
- ✓ Individuals who utilize nitrates, organic nitrites, and nitric oxide donors, particularly those who use nitrates for alleviating chest pain.

- ✓ People who have had a negative reaction to any medication, including Viagra.
- ✓ Men who have been advised to abstain from sexual activities to prevent or worsen cardiovascular disorders are being encouraged to lower their risk of cardiovascular complications.

Made in the USA
Las Vegas, NV
06 May 2024

89578668R10030